CONTENTS

FORWARD

When I look back, I can't believe my bad luck. I had just moved to a new city and was looking forward to new adventures. The morning of my car accident was full of bright sun and optimism. I was on my way to my new job, driving rather than taking the bus. After work I was meeting a real estate agent to look for a new home. Little did I know that this day would alter the rest of my life.

There is an old Chinese proverb that speaks to individual life events. When something happens do not assume immediately if it is good or bad; time will tell. There is still time in my life to tell a better story.

I write this book in the hope that others can find common ground; to know they are not alone. I have been dealt some mighty blows, yet I hold on to optimism. While my prior life is gone, maybe the new one will hold great surprises.

LIABILITY DISCLAIMER AND USER AGREEMENT

The content is not intended to be a substitute for professional medical advice, diagnosis, or treatment, and does not constitute medical or other professional advice. Reliance on any information provided herein is solely at your own risk.

State of being

(A personal poem)

Life is a state of being.

Being in the present.

Being at ease with your past.

Being who you are.

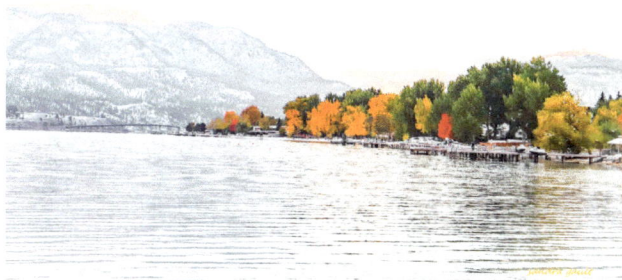

LIFE BEFORE

The morning of my car accident was warm and sunny. I was driving to work, and meeting a realtor after to search for a new home. I was in my new city for only two weeks, and I wondered about my place in the world. I struggled with the substance of my work and took a variety of courses to expand my thinking about meaningful work. I wanted to work with people, to do my part to make the world a better place. I could go on.

Emotions (A personal poem)

Everything – and nothing.

The storm is near.

Temptation and fear.

Madness and enlightenment.

Elusions of calm escape through the clouds.

Wind swept cliff beckon, and batter the fragile.

No loyalties are offered.

Only brisk winds remain.

THE BEGINNING OF THE END

I did not have any particular expectations for the future. Not fame; probably not fortune; but at least something meaningful. Traffic was nuts getting on to the freeway; I had to stop behind three other vehicles trying to merge. While watching traffic over my left shoulder I saw a flash of a white vehicle behind me, followed by my head flying forward and then back. In the flying forward motion, I felt my brain catch up to my skull, and a silent scream through my wide-open mouth.

My vehicle was mushed between two white vehicles. Consciousness (or whatever it was) was in slow motion. My side mirror was broken and the guy in the truck in front of me was getting out to check on me. I remember the ambulance worker asking if I had my seatbelt on (I had taken it off after the accident for some reason). In the ambulance the worker asked if I had blood pressure issues. What a stupid question! I was in shock. I don't remember the hospital at all. What I remember next was being in bed at my sister's and her phoning into work saying she had to keep an eye on her concussed sister.

Even in a terrible state of confusion, I remember the bedroom well. Odd to have such a monumental thing happen, and then feel confined in such a small space. Whether you had an accident or illness, you probably had a "what the hell happened" moment(s). Normal life – strike! Why couldn't I get my head off the pillow and why do I walk like I had way too much to drink? The next many years would become a blur.

Invasion of the body snatchers? Have you seen that movie called "The Man with 2 brains"? The scientist had a beautiful but bitchy wife. He fell in love with a brain in a jar and implanted the nice brain into the bitchy, beautiful body. Can I have that please?!

Here is the short list:

- concussion that caused dizziness for five years

- couldn't stand unsupported for 2 years

- dislocated hip that pulled on my sciatic

- soft tissue damage EVERYWHERE

- IT band damage that pulled my knee cap off centre

- terrible whiplash; no bend left in my neck

- TMJ (what is this pain in my jaw?)

- general anxiety, panicattacks, depression, PTSD......

SURVIVING FIBROMYALGIA

In the years that followed I worked harder, studied harder and was a social animal. Charity work was a passion and I gave and gave; of my time and funds. From the outside I might have appeared that I had a good life. It was, in part, a lie. I completed 3 more business certificates, and in my quiet revolt against my meaningless job, I took photographic design, darkroom developing, painting and others. I connected to a peace movement and continued my spiritually journey. I connected with a great group of friends for travel, along with a few family vacations with my sister and nephew. I refuse to give up! Having a full range of emotions, all at the same time, is confusing. Who am I mad at? Who I am I NOT mad at?! Anger is easier than sadness.

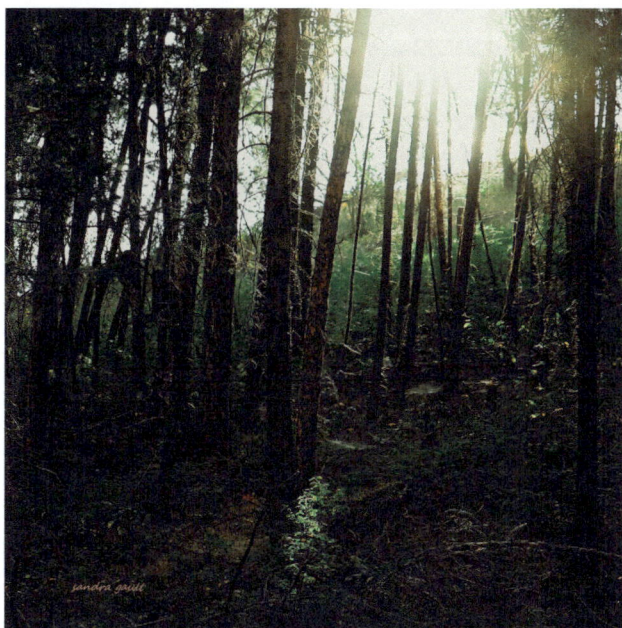

ACCEPTANCE

(Space for reflection)

Yikes! That's a HUGE ask, and one I will struggle with the rest of my life. Having others accept is also critically important. This includes loved ones, co-workers, society, and who else is important in your life.

What can you do for yourself (be a little selfish here) to feel/ be accepted?

EXHAUSTION AND WEIGHT GAIN

Did I sleep? I don't feel like it. I have muscles that hurt, where I didn't know there was a muscle. If I have a little caffeine or chocolate maybe my energy will increase. My favorite tea beverage isn't helping. I don't like coffee, so maybe more chocolate. Pure caffeine supplements make me jittery. Every day feels like the biggest struggle of my life! It has to get better, doesn't it????

Next day; no sleep again. I have always slept on my back. I tried sleeping on my side but the muscle spasms are horrible. There is no comfortable position. Night and day are melding into each other; I am always awake. My boss says I am doing well but my life is one big haze. Panic. Eventually my exhaustion become so extreme that I have blackouts at work. Being without benefits I work more than full days. I am awake so early that I go in hours before I need to, which of course is insanity. But I won't let it beat me and it keeps my mind off my so-called existence! The head injury is so severe that I have five years of dizziness and confusion in my surroundings.
I have no idea how I managed to use my intelligence when I was puzzled about everything else.

Most doctors do not know to treat chronic pain. Days and

weeks passing in the haze. I am eating all the time in an effort to feel energy in my body. Surprisingly I have lost 10 pounds in the first several months. I find out later that this is common as the body is working hard to heal. I always had enough energy to work, play sports, travel, to spend time with friends. I make an effort to spend some social time with coworkers. Eating out is part of the social scene, and I am enjoying it too much. Eventually the weight starts to pile on. My therapists tell me to concentrate on feeling better, and ignore the weight. Not good advice, because it NEVER comes off.

It is impossible to describe, to others, exhaustion so extreme it controls your life; every little bit of it! Is it the head injury, soft tissue damage from my knees to the top of my head? This HAS to get better. When the doctor cuts me off the sleeping pills, pain killers and muscle relaxers, all at once, life becomes impossible. I don't want to live if this is what life is. I go into a depression so deep I fear I will never come out. Hell is an individual in pain. I am too exhausted to worry about panic attacks and road rage created from the accident that ruined my life. I vaguely remember one day when I was in such a haze that I stood staring at the cross-walk light, not knowing what to do. I wanted to crawl under the covers, permanently. I barely slept for five years. Five years!

DOCTORS & PAIN MANAGEMENT (NOT!)

I had a GP that put me on pain, anti-inflammatories, and sleeping pills shortly after the accident. Regular physio-therapy, and massage therapy to start. I asked the physio-therapist for help with movement and balance issues. She referred me to a movement specialist. I needed to relearn how to walk, get out of a chair and bed properly again. Months after I was still picking my head off the pillow, while rolling the rest of my body out of bed. Did you know that an average human head weighs 10 pounds, and I have a big head. Lol. My sister used to laugh because a ski hat she got me for Christmas did not fit my "fat head". Full of brains I used to tell her. Good thing I have strong arms, as I needed them to push myself out of bed. After two years the GP refused to renew all my prescriptions. Her logic was that I should not continue on medications forever. What?! Down a deep, dark hole of depression I go. I don't like the term rabbit hole; rabbits are cute and I am not, anymore.

After six months, or more, my physio therapist said she could not help me any further. I was not improving. And she was a good therapist; I respected her. Each time I went for treatment she yanked my left leg to balance my dislocated left hip, and each visit it crawled back into the wrong spot (too much soft tissue damage pulling it out of place). My sciatic is being yanked on because of the hip dislocation. Oh fun! Being a flexible pretzel used to be fun. My physio pretzel manipulation was not amusing. Massage therapy is tricky. It hurts, it feels better for a few days, it hurts again. Hot stone massage is slightly relaxing, but I leave feeling unsatisfied.

For two years I could not stand unsupported. The insurance company tells me I will likely be followed by the other insurance company to confirm my injury state. That's creepy. I must have looked crazy hanging onto walls and the bus stop sign. The bus is like an exhibition ride; bump, bump, whirl. The physio therapist refers me to a movement specialist. Dislocated hip, no bend in neck, tissue damage everywhere. Getting out of a chair required a table or desk in front to push myself up. The movement specialist helped with standing, walking and general movement issues. I still walk like I am drunk, and I wobble when standing, but at least I am standing. That will change, just like the ebb and flow of life.

Acupuncture is an ancient practice, and I read it helps with a variety of ailments. I had treatment years ago for allergies and sinus pain.

I make an appointment with a naturopath that is now trained in the art/treatment. The long needles don't bother me; compared to the pretzel positions my physio therapist put me in. Why do I feel like throwing up? With every new needle the dizziness gets worse. Since the accident I notice increased sensitivity to the energy in and around me. I can feel the energy move from one needle meridian to the next like a super highway. Acupuncture is supposed to balance the Chi, the energy in the body, but I don't know if it is working because I spend the entire therapy sessions feeling sick. Disappointed in my body, again. Next.

There is a new Centre for Alternative Medicine downtown close to work. That is helpful as I use my lunch break to go for treatment. I receive nutrition advise on foods that may assist and worsen my tension and widespread pain. It becomes important that I avoid foods that cause inflammation. That's a long list; sugar, vegetable oils, refined carbs, alcohol and others. I pass on the acupuncture after a few sessions. Entrainment is a bio-musicological therapy that synchronizes organisms to a beat. I am given headphones, where in each ear there is a different conversation, and blinders. What? It puts me to sleep with no perceived benefits. At least I got a short nap in during the day. Bonus! I am grateful that someone is trying to help. Next!

I call the movement therapist to see if she has suggestions. She has a co-worker that does Craniosacral therapy. Cranio: head? Sacral?

I am still confused about the word, but it is energy work that releases tensions deep in the body to relieve pain and dysfunction. Again, I am very sensitive to energy work. I do feel some temporary relief, and I continue the treatment for some time, but again there is an invisible wall of pain that I can't move beyond. I am very disheartened. Actually...devastated. I take a reiki course to understand energy better. I can feel mine and others energy and blockages, but my back is too messed up to stand over another person in order to help them. I want to help me, and others. But how?

One thing at a time. One therapy at a time. My head hurts. Multi-tasking is becoming more and more challenging. I understand the terrible concussion and dizziness but what does that have to do with the pain in my jaw? I go to a dental specialist that tells me I have TMJ. Like everything in my body my jaw received damage. Damage aside I am told that stress contributes to the grinding of teeth at night. I am holding my whole body, my whole existence, stiff. Exercises to keep the teeth apart, and relax the jaw (relax?) don't work. I get dental trays full of goopy stuff shoved into my mouth for impressions. The mouthguard is supposed to reduce the tension and pain created by the nightly grinding. Not much help, and I gag when I put it in. There is a never-ending nightly search for the damn thing in the bed because I yanked it out during the night several times, unconsciously. Go fish! The jaw never went back into place. I HATE the damn mouthguard. Even with the mouthguard I have to get several crowns because I am grinding like mad.

Did you know human bites can be as bad as animal bites; averaging around 100 p.s.i.?!

I can't find a regular GP; a problem in the city. My first two GP's went on sick leave and there was no doctor to replace them. Walk-in clinics won't give pain killers or sleeping pills. I try everything in the drug store. Over the counter sleep aids work too well; I feel sleepy for hours after I get up. I get really frustrated when people tell me to take camomile or valerian to sleep. I need a heavy cast iron frying pan to the head to knock me out! Melatonin was not available on the market until some years later.

Good thing the brain can only detect so much pain at a time. Otherwise I would scream all day.

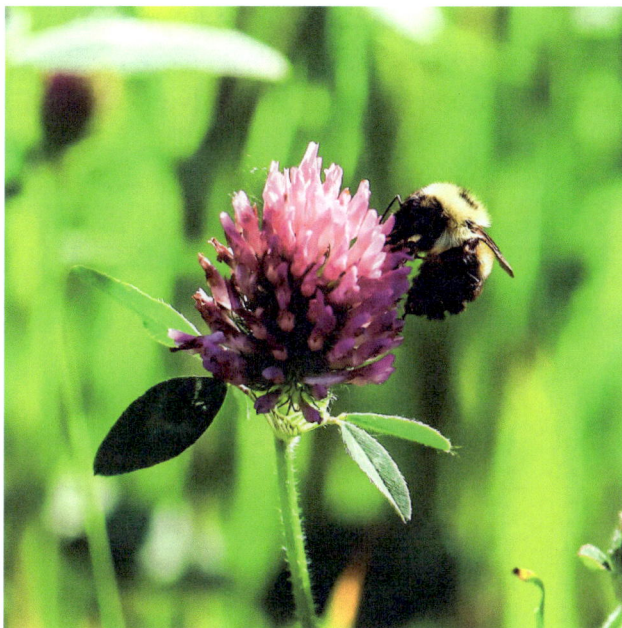

Take a break - Space for reflection

Sit quietly. Close your eyes, gently. Take slow breaths. Concentrating on the breath helps to keep you in the present. This is critical for well-being. Stress is created in the body and mind when you obsess over what was and what will be.

ALTERNATIVE/COMPLEMENTARY MEDICINE

Physio and massage therapy have been temporary help; I wish it were otherwise. And insurance only covers so much (so little). The amount of insurance coverage I have has not increased in 20 years, but I am grateful to have it. I need to regain my strength, movement and well-being. I was active my whole life; benefitted with a strong and flexible body. Thinking, praying, hoping there must be cures, I delve into the world of alternative treatments. It must have been Western doctors that coined that phrase. Complementary medicine works together with Western medicine (in my opinion), and can be very good for prevention.

Acupuncture – long needles and nausea. For temporary relief, and I can't afford the time or money to continue.

Entrainment – put me to sleep without any other benefit. My mind is crazy active with brain injury dizziness and an almost full body of pain and stiffness. How close can my shoulders get to my ears?

Active release – the bruises! Supposed to break down scar tissue but is too painful.

Movement retraining – at least got me moving somewhat better.

Craniosacral therapy – releases some tension. I am one of a small group that respond with active movement in therapy. I continue this for some time, but like every treatment, it does not get me beyond the high/extreme wall of pain.

Myofascial release – disturbing therapy where I relived some accident moments in my body.

Sound therapy – temporary relaxation.

Meditation – cannot sit up, so how can I concentrate/ not concentrate.

Chiropractor – temporary help with back tension.

Aromatherapy – smells good.

Reiki – I can feel energy moving, but it fails to unblock the pain.

Reflexology – relaxing, and I don't really like people working on my feet.

Spa day – I am not a person that enjoys being "pampered", and I don't like my nails painted. I want to have my muscle beat into submission.

Live blood testing – told me what already knew about my ailments, and did not provide suggested cures/relief.

Shockwave therapy – did help to reduce the golf ball sized muscle tension in my shoulders and upper back. Expensive though; insurance only covered a few sessions.

I am sure I have forgotten some. My family asks when I will give up. Ugh. Glad I kept my sense of humor…~~most~~ some of the time.

I hope you have better luck with therapy. There are a lot of wonderful practitioners.

Everything in the universe is swirling around at incredible speeds. Resist the temptation to control it.

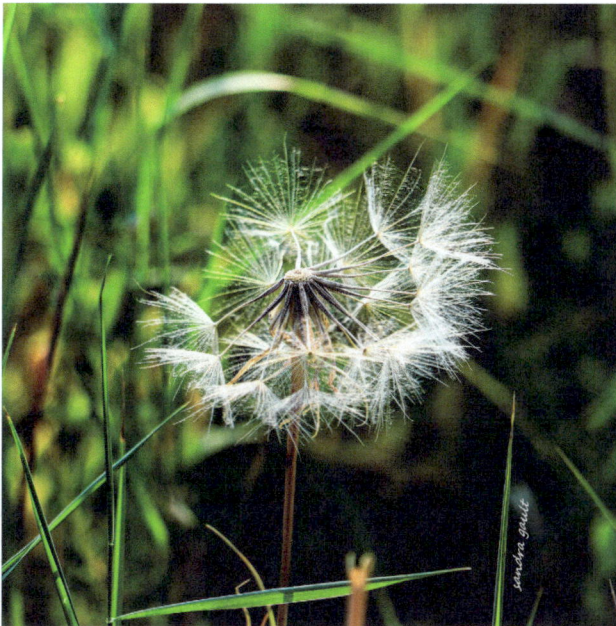

HERBS- SO MANY HERBS

A field of herbs is a lovely, relaxing vision. Healthy, tall growing green herbs gently swaying in the breeze. Ha!
Natural pain relievers can offer an alternative to long-term side effects of prescription pain medications. Ibuprofen is working great for inflammation and pain. And joy, they do not upset my stomach. Two decades later I learn that ibuprofen can cause serious health problems. I see a naturopath who does some testing and prescribes armfuls of herbs. Even they throw their arms up (I have too much to deal with). I start my own herbal research. I find it fascinating, but reading too much causes headaches. Here is a list of those I tried:

Valerian

5htp

Camomile

Bromelain

Magnesium

St john's wort

Ginseng

Bromelain

Flaxseed oil

Vitamin C

Ginger root

Milk thistle

Turmeric

Iodine

Probiotics

Turmeric

Oregano Oil

Lavender

Castor oil

B12 shots

Vitamin D

Homeopathy

Detox

I am not an expert, so I will not get into the purpose or dosage of these herbs. I don't find most of these as effective as relaxants or pain relievers, but it's better than the "nothing" I have from doctors. After years of experimentation and assistance from a knowledgeable friend and nutritional representative

I settle on a daily liver cleanse, B complex, magnesium, calcium, grape seed extract, Omega 3's, tumeric, plus meds of course.

I hope you do yourself the favor of being your own advocate when looking to feel better, and in every area of your life.

For my severe and widespread pain, I need more. I rely on handfuls of ibuprofen, acetaminophen, and herbs for many years. I am barely existing. If I could just have a good night sleep, I might feel better. Doctors tell me I might have healed better in the first five years if I had proper rest. As hard as I worked to feel better, I could not do it on my own. Everyone's story and needs and individual and personal. I felt rushed through the medical system; not very personal. It is challenging to feel heard; really heard.

You are more than your illness
- Space for reflection

Don't let judgement by others hurt. In all likelihood they are reacting out of fear and their own insecurities.

Remind yourself how wonderful you are! What strength you have! Go ahead! Boast!

MOVE?

Born with short, strong legs I played sports with my dad, sister, and friends. Dad taught me to ski, ride a bike and play tennis. I loved the fast-paced of tennis, racquetball, and downhill skiing. I also biked, ice skated, canoed, horseback riding, hiking, weight training, circuit training and golfing (not my fav, but I played with my parents).

After the accident I had no balance, no strength, and dizziness. Can't lean over bike handles without incredible pain, no balance to play fast sports, no coordination or energy to do any. Therapists say "move", but how? I can barely walk or stand straight. I do some push up, sit ups, and stretches, but I lack the energy to keep any exercise up. In the first few years when I was on enough meds to mask (or maybe blur) the chaos I tried to play tennis and golf again. Golf requires hip, leg and back rotation. Ouch! In tennis I felt like the ball rather than the hitter; but i don't bounce.

Being the "never give up" person I try many, more balanced exercises.

I enjoy Tai Chi (it is beautiful and meditative), but it requires too much coordination. Footwork is essential, and I do not know where my feet are. Beautiful to watch a group doing it outdoors.

Qigong is like a milder form of Tai Chi. The slow controlled movement feels good and it helps my balance a bit. My teacher has been doing it for decades.

Yoga is awesome. I like the fluid movements and meditative aspect. True to my love of strong, active exercise I lean towards power yoga. I do fairly well at it, especially due to my flexibility. I stick to it for a few years, but then comes the crash. Many years later (and after a ten-year absence) I find Hatha and Yin which are slow and restorative. More on that absence in life later.

Hard to describe Feldenkrais. It is a German method that consists of gentle, very slow, mindful movement. It is hard to move so slow, but is incredibly beneficial. After a series of 6 classes my teacher moves away.

I don't like the water so I avoided classes at the pool. Cold water, wet floors, common showers, yuck.

WORK HARD, PLAY HARD

I n the next ten or so years I live my life as best I can. Long hours and demanding work. I work in an industry that does not consider an individual's well-being. Bosses' attitudes are "burn em and churn em". I give it my all. I continue to study part-time, completing three more business certificates (project management, risk management and conflict management) and an industry trading/ marketing course. I do a lot of charity work; get voted into a corporate charity volunteer position, arrange fund raising, and other giving programs.

After too many years focusing on work- and work-related studies, I take several classes at the arts college; photographic design, dark room developing, Feng Shui, watercolor painting. How did my life get so focused on work? No wonder I can't relax! I also complete a program from a design school and become a professional organizer. I have always been clean and organized, not to mention a little OCD that runs in the family. Lol. If I start a part-time job helping people organize, I can carry that through into retirement. I love working with people and getting their mess organized will be fun and fulfilling.

Excessive work, work travel, pleasure travel, studies, going out with friends, no sleep, constant pain = burn out. My doctor tells me to be off work for six months. Being ridiculously dedicated I go back in 4, and feel sick every day for eight months. How many burn outs does it take to take you down? Not as many as I thought. After many years I sadly realized I was not going to get better; I thought I would go on one day at a time, struggling every moment, for the rest of my life. Such as it is.

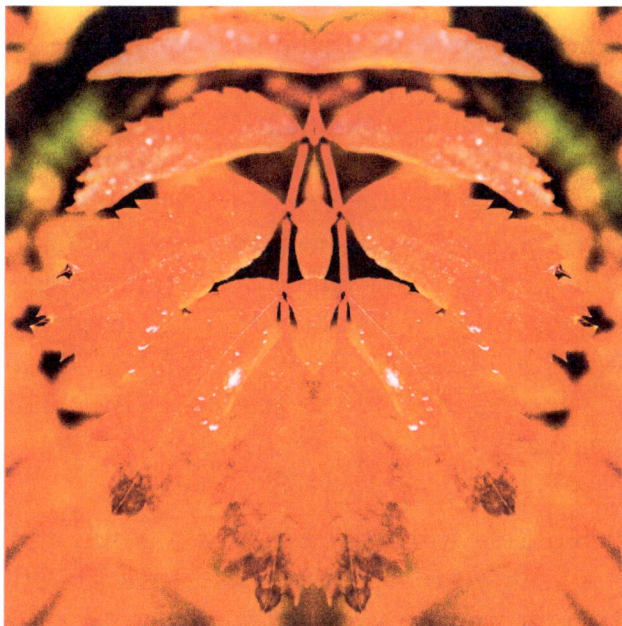

THE BIG CRASH

Approximately ten years after the accident I moved to a smaller city and company. It was closer to family and I hoped the work would not be so demanding. I desperately needed a balanced life (less work, more exercise, no more studying, more time outdoors where I always feel calmer). It was not to be. The job was equally demanding and while my first boss was wonderful, the second was a complete and abusive jerk. He did not care one bit about me and called me nasty names for no reason. And to top it off he was angry that I knew my job well and he didn't. He purposely embarrassed me at meetings to show his superiority. Really?! WTH?! They piled and piled the work on, running me into the ground...HARD. The beginning of the end!

The first building we worked in was modern and bright. After a few years we moved into an old, musty building that had sat empty for years. Allergies run in my family, and mine run to the environmental. The dreaded building was infested with mice, and was musty and smelly. I began to have worsening sinus congestion and pain.

I increased ibuprofen, general vitamins and decongestants. My allergist said the likely culprit, aside from the mice droppings, was black mold. The combination of the last burnout and musty building was lethal. Many other workers were having health problems, such as burning eyes and sore throat. I would feel better after the weekend and get progressively worse during the week. By Friday I was really sick. Hospital visits were becoming common, with terrible allergic reactions and weakness. The allergist was no help.

My last day at work was bizarre. I met a friend for an early lunch. Sitting at a nice outdoor table, I began to shake and fall over. My friend rushed me to the hospital. I couldn't walk, so she ran for a wheelchair. I was having convulsions. Doctors first thought it might be diabetic shock – I don't have diabetes. Blood tests, more tests, an assessment from the neurologist; they did not know the cause. They rule out Lyme disease and others. My explanation of allergic response did not resonate with the doctors. They send me home in a few days. I need a wheelchair. Did they drug me?

NEW SYMPTOMS, EVERY WEEK

I must be dying! But of what. I had to crawl from the bed to the couch. I am barely existing!

Here are some of the notes I made when new, severe symptoms, developed:

Severe rash and welts from my regular skin cream on neck and chin. Antibiotics and cortisone cream to help. Takes 5 days to clear up.

Another rash and swelling on face and neck. I watched the swelling as in minutes my forehead was so swollen, I could barely see. My immune system was crashing. Doctor gave me prednisone; again, and again. The pharmacist looked at me with sad expression.

Severe headaches and dizziness from reading for a short period. Strange rapid eye movement, in the left eye, and it felt like the side of my head was going to blow off. I don't expect to wake up the next day.

After two nights of barely sleeping due to these symptoms, in addition to shaking and weakness, I go to the hospital. After a five hour wait the doctor made note of head pain, dizziness, rapid heartbeat, weakness, rapid eye movement and shaking. Meds were given for headache and to slow heartbeat. I leave feeling not much better. I am weak and falling down.

Problems with numbers (adding up and reading).

Extreme weakness and shaking.

Worsening dizzy spells. Now getting black-outs.

New chiropractor detected anomalies in energy patterns in my head while reading. He has been reading about research in this area. He begins to help nerve flow to those areas.

Can't focus on hanging on to things. Or is it weakness?

After a short visit with a good friend I have complete exhaustion, headaches and upset stomach. I am popping a lot of anti-nauseants.

Got freaked out by an unusual commercial on TV. Things moving too fast freak me out.

Cold chills day and night for two weekbecome frightening. I can't make sense of my surroundings.

Panic attacks when I attempt to read my mail because I don't understand what I am reading. Words and sentences don't make sense. Is this a different language?

Short shopping trips cause severe headache, dizziness, shakes and confusion. Reading food labels, too many people, and bright lights are unbearable. Hanging onto the store cart for dear life. I fear it will tip over from putting so much weight on it; breaking my teeth.

Exhaustion so bad I can barely walk and stand. Blackouts when I am exhausted and need to rest. Why am I no better after sleeping 18 hours? I ask my doctor for a disabled parking placard. I am embarrassed to use it.

Got lost on a familiar road. Did not know how to get home and had a major panic attack (I was five blocks from home and did not recognize anything).

Major mental breakdown when I am denied disability benefits (have been off work for 6 months at this point).

Still getting bad earaches, especially on the left side. These started 6 months before the collapse. What is with all the left side stuff: headaches, earaches, dislocated hip, numbness down left side from hip.

I am afraid to leave the house.

Numbness in finger on right hand. It is starting to spread to other fingers and the hand.

So weak, getting on and off toilet is almost impossible. I need the counter to pull myself up.

Burning and pain in right arm is increasing. Numbness has increased to all fingers on both hands.

Scared to drive because it feels like cars are rushing by at warp speed.

When I am able to get into the shower, I get stuck inside because I am too weak to open the door. Even if I scream, no one will hear me.

In the movie 3 Men and a Baby they have a phone installed in the shower. Good idea.

Sleeping longer and longer; about 11 hours a night now, plus naps.

Legs and total body shaking and weak. Almost impossible to walk. Friends have to help me, when they are around.

Burning in feet really, really painful. What are they burning from?

Some numbness in lips. Is it another allergic reaction?

Dropping things all day. Placing items in wrong places. A lot of confusion.

When I turn sideways I blackout. Cooking is impossible.

Increased difficulty writing. Filing out medical forms requires assistance.

Dull and then shooting pain in both feet and legs. Can't sleep.

Numbness is moving up into my legs from the feet.

Writing almost impossible. Even signing my name.

Bad skin breakouts all over face. My face has always broken out when under stress but this is crazy.

Skin so sensitive, putting on lotion and clothing hurts. Fleece is soft. I live in pj's. It's okay to answer the door in pj's, isn't it? I did put on a hoodie.

Short-term memory is still very poor. Some long-term

memory coming back. Good thing I am keeping records of what's been going on.

Tried to read after a long avoidance. Still getting wicked headaches and nausea.

Some days my feet stop moving and I have to stand still for a time. It happens in parking lots a lot when I get out of the car. I stare at my feet, but I can't tell them to move. It's easier to not look at them.

Can only sit up for short periods. I lay on the couch for long periods and watch birds sail by.

I am embarrassed that I cannot understand conversations, or speak without slurring.

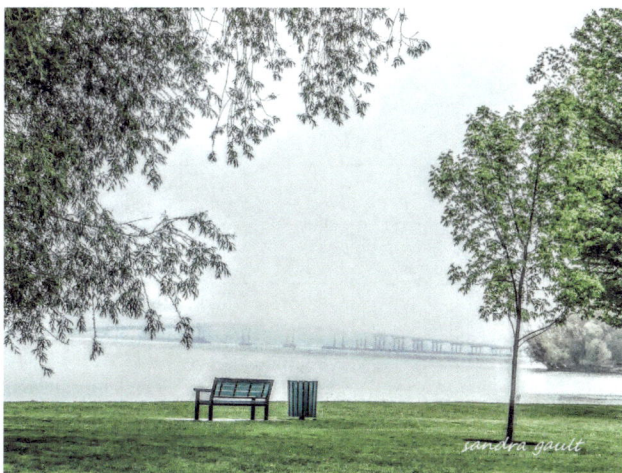

Self care is critical -
Space for reflection

You do not have to do everything you did before. Seriously. Rest when you need to. Ditch the guilt.

What can you do for yourself to decompress?

I HAVE LOST EVERYTHING

My life was: work, learning, reading, traveling, sports, volunteering, social coordinator, laughing, dreaming, time with family, movies, walking, camping.... I loved to try new things. Flying lessons, rode a camel on the Sahara Desert, parasailing over the Indian Ocean, ziplining, hiking way up in the mountains, white water rafting, whale watching, sailing, downhill skiing through slalom poles, weight training. And I loved to stretch my imagination and intelligence; reiki training, art classes, calligraphy, ancient philosophy, history, ancient symbols, Eastern and Western early thought, art history, science, architecture. I had a thirst for knowledge and a great imagination. I believe anything is possible in the universe and felt my connection with it.

Can't walk, work, shop, cook, clean, travel, drive, talk, read, think, laugh, be.

Lost my super-human abilities; great strength, always knowing north, intelligence (I understood everything

I read, including very technical), equally right and left brained, ambidextrous, reading upside down as fast as right side up, mathematical and spiritual, balance and co-ordination for sports. I had all my confidence removed. I was nothing.

Everything is very confusing. I am in such a fog that life doesn't even feel real. I am falling over all the time. And the blackouts; even when I turn my head sideways to pick something up. Watching TV is strange; when something moves fast my brain fails to understand, and I get scared, really scared. It makes me feel as if I am an alien watching TV, and the world in general. This makes cooking impossible. Friends and family bring me food sometimes. My legs buckle underneath me constantly.

There needs to be more railings and things to hang onto. Getting caught on the toilet with no strength to get up is frightening. When not crawling from the bed to the couch (good thing I have a small apartment), I hang onto the wall. When the wall ends, I panic on how I am going to get anywhere. I never got lost in a foreign country; now I lose everything, including road layouts in my home town, everything in the house, and I don't understand the layout of clock hands. How do I go downstairs to get the mail? Will people think I am nuts if I get the mail in my pj's? When I do get the mail, I don't understand what I am reading. Numbers make no sense; I can't understand my bills.

I need a piece of paper to add simple numbers now. Good thing I have most expenses set up for automatic withdrawal.

I hate to depend on friends and family so much, so I take a cab sometimes to get groceries and to get to appointments. I wonder every time I sleep if I am going to wake up. I am sleeping on average 18 to 20 hours a day.

When surviving minute to minute is impossible, there are no thoughts of things to do, life outside the apartment, and essentially the rest of the world. I was always a very active, focused, dedicated, intelligent person. I can't even think about a normal life.

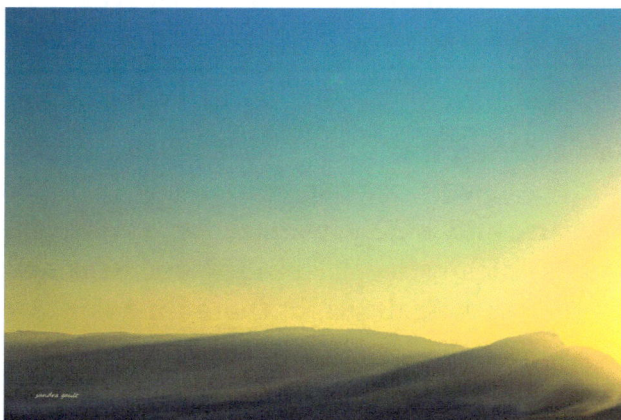

The devastation was extreme:

Can never work again because I do not understand numbers and I can't be upright for very long. An hour of lunching with friends or family means a two-hour nap; at least. My disability benefits are such that if I am unable to volunteer, even for an hour. What a ridiculous and thoughtless rule! Not that I have the energy to volunteer anymore. I have never felt that I have done enough in the world to help others; to be a good citizen of the world; a friend to nature and animals. When you are barely surviving helping others is not possible, but the guilt is always there.

I could not read anything for five years after the crash; not even emails or my mail. I needed help doing my taxes and thank goodness my friend is my financial advisor because I do not understand the statements. My life long love of reading (researching for work and reading fiction and non-fiction) was yanked from me. I understood words, but not sentences. I felt like a needy child, in an adult body.

When stressed from life I have always taken a walk in nature. I was almost completely bed-ridden for two years, and barely walked for 5 after that. Getting a handicap sticker from the doctor is depressing and embarrassing. It's right there…in your face. Ugh. I often could not make it into the store, let alone shop. Friends helped me to and from the car when meeting for coffee. Walls are my friend; I cannot stand unsupported for more than a few minutes. Traveling would be gone FOREVER!

Can't cook. Can't walk around a store or stand at the checkout without almost collapsing. I have scary visions of blackouts in the line at Walmart! That picture would probably show up on someone's Facebook. Can't get the fridge door open. Can't stand at the counter. Can't turn sideways to grab a utensil. Can't remember recipes! From the time I could crawl on the stool next to counter I wanted to help cook. By the time I was in grade 2 I was able to cook a meal for the whole family.

I even helped my older sister who was at a loss in the kitchen. That still makes me laugh about the day she was "trying" to make rice on the stove. She did not measure the water and rice, so the rice was swimming. I don't know how long she was staring at it. I instructed her to pour off the water, place the rice in a microwave safe bowl and try to cook off the excess moisture. A while later I returned to the kitchen to find she had not drained the water and was staring at the microwave like it was a TV! OMG!

I felt like a dunce. Brain fog and injury, numbness in my face and partially in my tongue, meant I had to talk slow. But I can barely think of what I want to say, let alone say it. I was born with confidence to speak in front of anyone. At my company I was told I was the best public speaker. In a casual setting I spoke with intelligence and wit. Spoke; past tense. When did I become dumb? I cannot focus on anything or anyone, I wanted to hide from the world. I had the best excuse; I was barely able to get out of the house.

Money problems. The freaking icing on the cake as one may say? Because of my dedication to my company, and the fact that I did not currently have disability insurance when I had my car accident I continued to work. Every day it was "I can't do it", and everyday I did more. I got almost nothing from insurance because I kept working. My lawyer did not tell me this would happen.

A specialist said by the time I would turn 60 I would have fibromyalgia and will be disabled. She was spot on; and still I got almost nothing.

I used that little bit of money on alternative therapies within 3 years; ever searching for "the cure". When I moved to my current city 15 years ago, I took a 30% cut in pay to be close to my family. When put on disability I lost another 33% in income. Yes, happy to have disability, but crap! And here is the icing; I met and married a narcissist who cheated me out of a pile of money. What is left is so little I am stuck in a tiny apartment. NOT HAPPY! When I hit retirement age, I lose even more money as I did not work for long enough to save enough. This is not good for my peace of mind for the future, and my need to have peace and quiet.

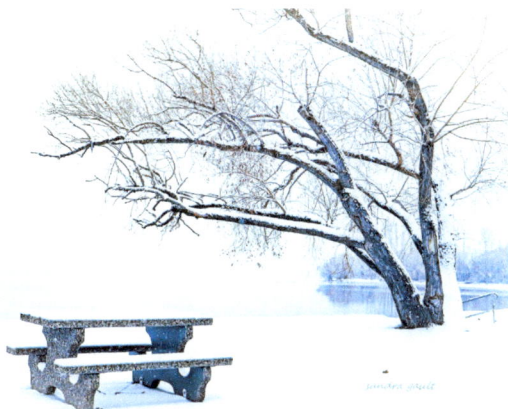

12 SPECIALISTS + TESTS + MEDS

My barrage of symptoms are nothing short of punishing. My GP was convinced it was another work burnout. It wasn't. I had to tell her that again and again. After many visits (what is that nice word being used for such an unpleasant thing) to the hospital, the third neurologist has a theory. His diagnosis: brain injury! I make an appoint to see my GP, excited (?) that we have somewhere to go, and she refused to look at the neurologist report. WTH! She stood firm on her original diagnosis of burnout and depression. She is adding to my depression.

Weeks of no miraculous recovery spread into months. What am I to do?! I keep telling my job "another few weeks and I will be back to work". My mom panics and says to hurry my doctor for a diagnosis because I have to get back to work. Friends don't know what to think. I go to a walk-in clinic and the doctor there says I have all the signs of a stroke. After a trip to the hospital; it's not. I look for a new GP. I interviewed with a few who said my case is too confusing and won't take me as a patient.

I get more frightened and depressed. I am not depressed; I am living a nightmare. Other doctors I see in the future note my "sunny disposition", especially considering my symptoms. I look up my weirdness regarding getting lost, problems reading and general brain problems. I find one particularly useful chart that sets out the area that feels it is going to explode when reading, it is the cognitive centre. That makes sense?! Left brain, behind and above the ear is responsible for language, special arrangement of language, math skills, reading clocks! Reading clocks?! That's weird. It says that on the chart. Was I meant to find that chart? There I go thinking of fate again.

Not being able to find help in a new GP, I made strategic plans for visits with my current GP. I took the worst of the symptoms, one at a time, and presented the problem to her. First on the list was dizziness. Was there a specialist that could provide some insight? Yes, there is a Vestibular Therapist in town. Good. This therapy uses specialized exercises for sight and walking/balancing stabilization. After some testing and exercises I was not improving. The diagnosis was severe dizziness with "unknown" cause. Not vertigo.

Naturopaths are so valuable for health and prevention. Lab tests included urinalysis, blood work and saliva and allergy testing. I saw two and got the same diagnosis; adrenal and chronic fatigue. They try to explain, but my now seemingly smaller brain barely understands.

From my limited understanding adrenal fatigue stems from exhaustion and the body being unable to produce adequate quantities of hormones and cortisol. This can happen from chronic stress or infections. Signs are low energy, trouble sleeping, weight gain, mood swings, depression, anxiety, brain fog, low absorption of food nutrients, and autoimmune issues. Yup. Have all of those. But how to treat? Lots of nutrients. Huh?! A friend introduces me to a friend that has great knowledge on nutrients. Great. This new friend provides some articles and information and we get going on some problem solving. We are still tweaking, and still friends.

My optometrist is a great guy. Maybe he will have some insight on the dizziness? I take a list of issues and have a full exam. No abnormalities seen. Worth a try. My dizziness is making me dizzy. And, no...I am NOT a blond. Sorry to the blonds...that was insulting.

I ask my doctor to refer me for an MRI. She refuses, given that she still thinks I am just tired and depressed. Arg! Even in my disastrous state I understand I am not those things. I go back, telling her that I will pay for it. My need to understand my sick brain is of utmost importance to me. She gives me the requisition. I have small canals to my ears, and the pressure created from the plugs creates enormous pressure. They try several pair; they can't get the left one to stay in. They put headphones on top. That works okay. Results come a few days later.

No abnormalities on the brain. Oh! It was just the brain I was having done.

Allergies run in my family. In 2008, after a bad work burnout, I never felt well. While my doctor gave me orders not to work overtime, my boss thought otherwise. I fought him to no avail. My immune system was challenged and when we moved into a moldy office building, I was quickly inundated with severe sinus headaches, respiratory issues, burning eyes nose and throat, coughing, weakness, congestion, throat constriction. Many hospital trips with severe allergic reactions; weakness, difficulty walking and talking, labored breathing, and convulsions. The hospital each time gave me a strong antihistamine and medication to ease my breathing and rapid heartbeat. One hospital doctor noted my allergic reaction to be severe, with unusual neurological symptoms.

I have been seeing an allergist for years. They do extra testing and come up with a black mold reason for the symptoms. Black mold, as I was to understand, is almost impossible to locate and get rid of. My boss screamed at me again and again for being ill, telling me my allergist is responsible for determining how to get rid of the problem in the office. Three doctors notes to stay out of the mold office are disregarded by my boss. This is the beginning of the end of my work career.

All that dedication and studying! Twenty years of part-time studies and 30 years of work!

My company recently hired disability specialists to get employees back to work. I go for a meeting and am threatened. Two people stood over me telling me I needed to sign my rights away to doctor and hospital medical records. Next time I take a union rep and they are sweet as pie. I am required to do some testing to determine my ability to do any work. I can't sit or read! Numbers don't make sense anymore. I am so exhausted and stressed that I need help to get into a cab. Another part of the requirements is to see their psychologist. He has no empathy. In the first session he tells me I am too old to have childhood issues. Everyone I know has them! He was, however, able to give a diagnosis of stress and post traumatic stress from being severely ill. The diagnosis was based on my fears of death, loss of confidence, fear of the future, and feeling defeated and hopeless.

I write this desperate note to my GP for help:

Over the past few years have been hard, distressing and painful. I have a very busy stressful job where I was forced to work an excessive number of hours under extreme stress and abuse. In 2008 I was physically and mentally exhausted and took 2 ½ months of bed rest. I never recovered from this exhaustion and it continued and worsened.

The company I work for is extremely hard on its employees and there are firings and blame thrown around when it is often unwarranted.

Throughout the period from 2008 to 2010 my health and immune system continued to decline, reaching the breaking point in 2010 when I was hospitalized and bed ridden. My disability and symptoms are so severe that I have had nightmares that I am dying from my conditions. I am barely able to read and walk, don't understand most of what I do read, have terrible dizziness and weakness, get lost on familiar streets, and have been almost unable to look after myself (cooking, cleaning, grocery shopping, getting to appointments etc.).

During the past eight months that I have been off work I have received threats from my company and the rehabilitation company that works for them, adding to my stressful situation. At one point I had not received any income for three months. I am not getting better and I fear I do not have a future. I get out and spend as much time with friends and family as I am capable, but it is challenging to keep any optimism that things will improve and that I will one day have a normal life again. I am doing all I can to understand what is wrong and have sought out many medical practitioners for help.

I am at a loss as to how to move forward, and my exhaustion, dizziness and other physical symptoms are limiting my ability to do the basic necessities of life.

Over the past month I have developed severe panic attacks when I get lost or read something and don't understand. In 2011 I was denied long-term disability by the insurance company and had a severe mental breakdown. I have had many years of excruciating physical and emotional stress and am open to any suggestions from my doctors for getting my life back on track. I feel desperate and lost.

Chiropractic is a health field I don't really understand, but was willing to try. My lovely chiropractor does ex-rays, tests and an exam. Ex-rays show I have no bend left in my neck. The result of severe whiplash. Soft tissue damage from my knees to my head, dislocated hip etc. is causing some spinal issues (the muscles are pulling my body structure out of allignment). Diagnosis: Spinal decay, postural distortions and nerve stress. I have issues in 1C, 2C, 3C, 7C, 1Tand 2T. These affect blood supply to the head, neck muscles, shoulders, thyroid, lower back, sciatic, heart and lungs. The effects of which are insomnia, headaches, dizziness, chronic tiredness, stiff neck, pain in upper arm, backache, sciatica. The weekly adjustments are a little helpful and I continue for some time.

This chiropractor in addition was researching how reading can cause dizziness and head pain. He tries a few procedures, with limited success.

A friend tells me about a neuro-psychologist in town. Neuro what? My doctor provides a referral. They evaluate and treat people with various types of nervous system disorders, illnesses, injuries and diseases of the brain, and how these affect the way a person feels, thinks and behaves. Numbers don't make sense. I have brain fog to the extreme and mass confusion. I must have come across like a nut job! It is uneasy sitting across from an expert who is evaluating your every word and movement. The assessments were supposed to take a week, but I am unable to be there more than an hour or so at a time. I don't know what to expect, and I only vaguely remember the tests. A series of remembering numbers, shapes, words, short sentences. I never saw the final report, but he did report functional and structural problems in my brain, in terms of cognition, attention, memory, language.I believe cognitive disfunction was the term.

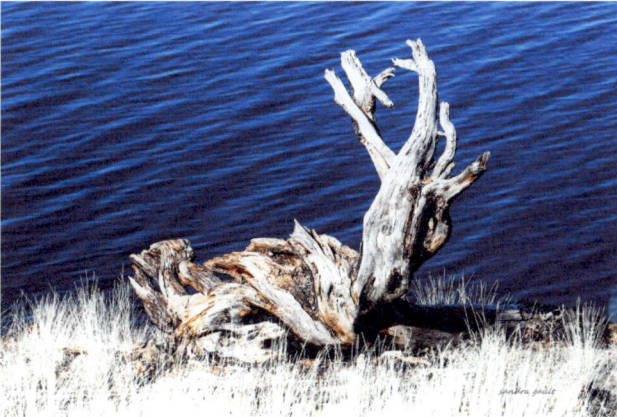

Don't give up! - Space for reflection

There is hope. There is help. Ask for help. It is NOT a weakness.

Remind yourself of the wonderful blessings you have in your life.

FINALLY, A DIAGNOSIS

Oddly enough it was the last, severe symptom that led to the diagnosis. Shooting pain in legs and feet is excruciating. Nerve conduction testing at the hospital by a rheumatologist reveals that there is no nerve issue in my legs and feet. This is the 12th doctor I have seen in the past 10 months. To each doctor/specialist I take a list of symptoms and other specialists seen; the list is long. The doctor doing nerve conduction testing is not very personable but he is the key. He reviews my history and long list and tells me; "You do not have nerve conduction problems, but I know what you do have; I have seen many such patients. You have fibromyalgia. "Join a support group, take medication and live the best life you are able." He was spot on!

Doctor doesn't believe diagnosis

I did the work that led to the diagnosis. My doctor rarely went along with my requests. It was ten months of exhausting tests and frightening symptoms. I had heard of people dying while they are waiting for a diagnosis. My own grandmother and cousin died because the diagnosis came too late. I expected that I would fall to the same fate. My doctor was no help. She wrote me off at the beginning.

In her defence, my list of symptoms was unbelievable. Or was it? I look up fibromyalgia on the internet (thank goodness for my new tablet, as I can't sit at the desk). I show up at my doctor's office, somewhat happy, as I was not currently dying. I am met with great scepticism. She sends a report to my insurance company that I have severe depression and work burnout, and don't know what else.

It takes me a while before I grasp why she may have that diagnosis; I was not her patient when I had my car accident, and for many years after. I prepare a short medical history for her:

Age 34: Bad car accident – rear ended. Bad concussion, whiplash, dislocated left hip due to muscle damage, extensive soft tissue damage. Had physiotherapy, massage therapy, acupuncture, movement retraining, cranial sacral therapy and others. Dizziness for five years. Could not stand unsupported for two years. Continue to have extensive chronic muscle pain in many areas from knees to neck.

3 years ago: Burnout caused me to be off work for two months and returned to work gradually over the third month.

Doctor suggested I be off work for six months but due to pressure from work I returned earlier. Had excessive exhaustion and illness for about eight months after returning to work.

The next 2 years: Burnout continued and worsened. Each time even a few hours overtime or otherwise busy life or minor illness such as cold and flu, burnout worsened and did not improve. Almost unable to continue normal activities any day of the week. Allergies (severe sinus headaches, respiratory issues, burning eyes, nose and throat, coughing, weakness, congestion, throat constriction) worsened considerably and I had to be moved to another work location due to worsening allergic response and general health. Allergist suggests it may be a mold issue in the one work location. Several visits to the allergist did not determine the problem (there are no tests for respiratory allergic response to molds and others).

Starting 6 months before my crash: Had serious allergic reaction from meeting at old work location. Went to hospital with extreme weakness and difficulty walking, difficulty breathing, tight chest, wheezing, sinus pain and discharge and convulsions. Each time I was forced to return to the problem building the allergic response came faster and harder. Allergy turned to toxic shock, and triggered severe fibromyalgia symptoms.

The toxic shock connection came from a small book in the pharmacy that I happened upon by chance(?) one day. It was written by an American allergy specialist.

My doctor had the "ah ha" moment and finally agreed with the diagnosis from the rheumatologist.

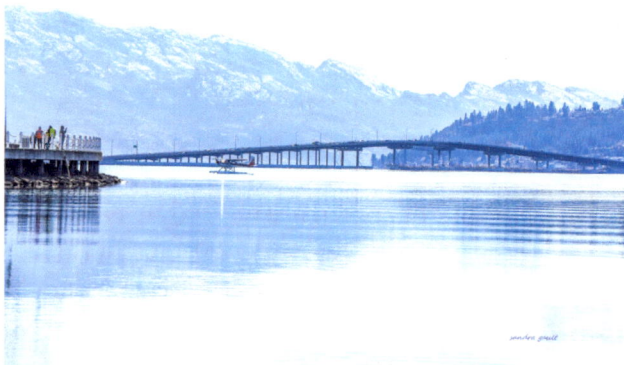

GET TO KNOW YOUR ILLNESS

I found a course that ran once a week, for 2 hours each class, on Fibromyalgia at the local Arthritis Society. My doctor provides a recommendation. The classes started about a year after my collapse, and I was still in a terrible fog. I attended the classes, but was unable to read the handouts. Our teacher was a physiotherapist, who specializes in arthritis and fibromyalgia patients. Thankfully he was thorough and understandable, and the best quality... a sense of humor. The funniest suggestions were, making a tent for your feet to keep blanket pressure off, wear headphones, blinders, and a hat and mitts if your extremities get cold. We roared at the insane visualizations.

Common fibromyalgia symptoms include:

Pain and tender points, debilitating fatigue, sleep problems, concentration and memory problems (fibro fog), anxiety, depression, widespread pain, deep pain, throbbing, aching, numbness, tingling in hands, arms, feet and legs, headaches, irritable bowel, urination problems. Where does the list end? Regrettably, it does not explain all my symptoms. How is that possible?!

Treatments include drugs, alternative remedies, and life-style habits. No cure. Antidepressants may help with pain, fatigue, depression, and anxiety. Pain relievers, muscle relaxants, anxiety drugs, and neuropathic pain pills. Physical therapy, moist heat, relaxation, and stress reduction. Hah! I'm sick! My life has fallen completely apart! Stress reduction?!

Let people in your life know that you have an illness that causes pain, fatigue, concentration and thinking problems.

- Listen to your body.

- Go to bed and wake up at the same time every day.

- Develop a relaxing bedtime routine, like a warm bath or reading.

- Make your bedroom beneficial to sleep by keeping   it dark and free of distractions like the TV and computer.

- Make time every day to decompress and relax.

- Do something you love like reading, listening to music, or taking a walk.

- Try meditation, massage or deep-breathing exercises to de-stress.

- Conserve energy. Cut back on less important things.

- Learn to say no.- Break down tasks into manageable bits.

- Try to get some gentle exercise. Work with a physio therapist if required.

After the six-week course I work with the physio therapist that taught the class. He does a walking assessment, then tries to teach me to walk with canes or walking poles. That makes walking impossible, as I can't coordinate my feet, let alone anything else. He tells me I have a disorder where I don't recognize my hands and feet. Is it because I have numbness in my fingers, toes, and left leg from my hip down? Numbness may be from the massive damage to my neck. I never know where that thing is supposed to be, because it doesn't sit properly on my shoulders anymore! Lol.

Neuropathy is where your extremities feel like they are tingling, burning, itching, shooting, or like ants are crawling on you. All of the above. So annoying and kind of yucky to think something is crawling on you. It's like camping, when you think you might have forgotten to close the tent and wonder what bugs might have made a home in your sleeping bag. Ewww! It also makes the skin sensitive to light touch of clothing or bedsheets on the legs. My feet have always been sensitive to tight sheets. I have now ditched the top sheet and have light coverlets instead of a heavy comforter.

Socks have never fit me because I have small feet. Now the sock problem is that I need to have loose ones that don't have stitching on the toes that will get irritating.; especially in shoes. Shoes! I have always felt more comfortable barefoot. Shoes with good arch support and comfortable, breathable material is what my feet feel the most comfortable in. Shoes with laces can also irritate.

Touching one finger to the next on one hand is massively confusing. That explains why I drop so many things. I think I had that test at the neuro-psychologist as well. It's a brain problem, caused by the car accident. I am sure the fibromyalgia and chronic fatigue add to it. I give up my nice stoneware dishes for light ones that don't break. I switch my water glasses to glass mugs that have handles. I feel my fingers tightening on the handle whereas a regular glass always feels like it is going to skip. I feel like I need to child proof my life. My poor brain doesn't know what to do. That's disturbing. I am too exhausted to go for physio therapy, so I give up, for now.

A few years later I work with another physio therapist, with the hope I can get better balance. I walk, I wobble like I am drunk, I bang into walls. I took a cruise many years ago, and a few nights on more open seas the ship was rocking so much that at one minute you were on one side of the aisle and the next on the other side. Want to dance? The therapist thinks my main problem is general weakness. She gives me some supported strength exercises.

I am not sure they are working and I am frustrated; I played a lot of sports and gentle exercises seem useless, but I keep at it. A few weeks later my regular therapist is away and the other therapist tells me I am not doing the exercises to the full extent. Really?! I tell her my regular therapist was happy with my workouts. She doesn't care. She pushes me hard, like I am training for a triathlon. I don't go back.

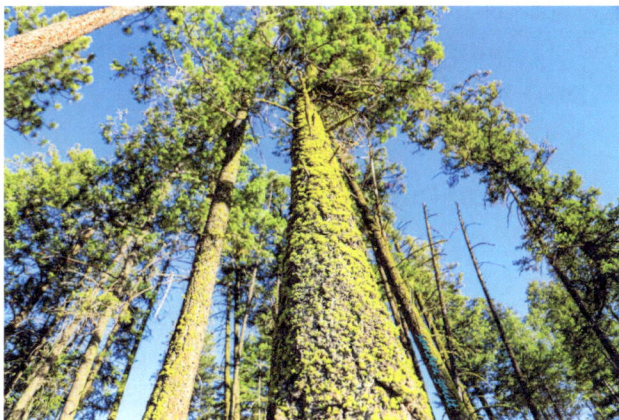

Different, but the same -

Space for reflection

I have/had some unusual symptoms. But from most people I have interacted with, there are a large number of common symptoms. Keeping track of those symptoms, for me, was critical in getting a diagnosis.

What are your symptoms?

CHRONIC FATIGUE SYNDROME

My GP writes an update to the insurance company that I also have chronic fatigue. For years I thought it was part of the fibromyalgia. When I finally do read about it, it helps to explain a bunch of other symptoms I can't make sense of. Chronic fatigue is a debilitating disorder with persistent fatigue that is not improved with rest. I can only sit up for so long before I have to lay down. I don't feel comfortable or rested sitting up. So, I have two separate illnesses that make me exhausted? I friend tells me to look of M.E. I think it's the same thing.

Chronic fatigue has neurological, immunological, and endocrine system irregularities (I copied that from somewhere as I am still unsure what it means). How can being exhausted be a nervous system disease? Did I get it from the years of overworking and studying after my car accident, when the fibromyalgia actually started? I told myself I was just living my life, but I may have been making matters worse. To live your life or not? That is a sucky and depressing decision.

I thought the car accident would leave me in pain for life, but WTH are the other symptoms doing in my body? Like fibromyalgia the possible symptoms are daunting:

- unrefreshing sleep

- widespread muscle and joint pain

- cognitive difficulties

- chronic, severe, mental and physical exhaustion

- muscle weakness

- hypersensitivity

- intolerance to sitting upright

- digestive disturbances

- depression

- immune system problems

- cardiac and respiratory problems

My quality of life has radically changed from the combination of fibromyalgia and chronic fatigue. And then there is my brain injury. A triple threat. I am exhausted from being exhausted; every molecule. Try to walk when you are weak, have numbness in feet and up the left leg to the hip, dizziness, soft tissue damage from the knees up, and a dislocated left hip. Needless to say, I will not be running any marathons! Feet temperature runs from the formerly hot, to cold. As you know how I hate socks! So, it's socks on, slippers on, slippers off, socks off...and repeat. Also explains the dropsies.

Am I having a stroke when my hand suddenly releases an object? It almost feels like a mini blackout (I have lots and lots of those). A combination of lack of mental connection to my fingers and toes, dizziness, blackouts, nerve damage, lack of concentration? So many things going on I must seem crazy when trying to explain to someone else. I am not myself. Am I someone new now?

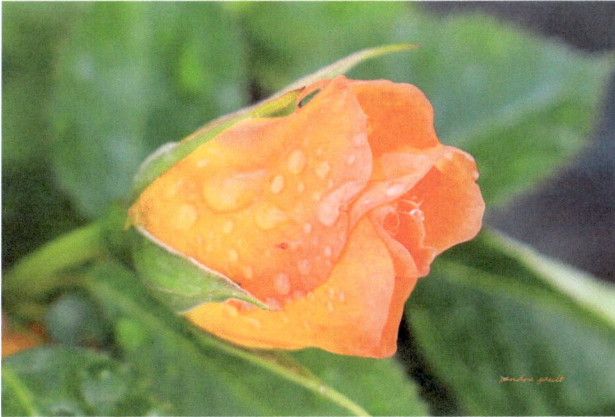

MEDS

Pile on the meds! It makes sense to go for the ones that are best known for fibromyalgia and chronic fatigue. After my accident there was little known about fibromyalgia and no doctors (that I knew of) that specialized in chronic pain. I was, initially, denied disability benefit because I had burnout and depression and who knows what else. Did you know that persons with chronic pain have shortened life expectancy? We were written off as depressed individuals. I was, until I fought for an answer. One well known med caused a fever, severe headache, vomiting and diarrhea. I cringe watching commercials where the cure is worse than the disease; may cause hair loss, incontinence, and death! I have some of the "if you develop these symptoms call a doctor immediately" reactions. One med is forced on me twice. I was labeled as difficult by my GP.

My search for a new GP took years. Many did not want to deal with a new patient with a complicated and severe medical history. How sad is that?! When you need one most, they push you out the door! When I finally get a new, great one we worked to get me feeling better.
He said it helped when I told him the "we" need to work together to get me better. New meds and changes in dosage are continuous as the degree of symptoms transform over

the years. Recently a group of pain clinic therapists tell me it is all in my head. They stated categorically that my emotions are causing the pain. They say "don't you feel better when you are in a good mood"? No!!! I feel the same all day and night. If I toss and turn my back pain is really bad for the next few days. Light stretching helps a bit. It is so crazy that the thing I need is sleep but I am so messed up I cannot sleep without a lot of help.

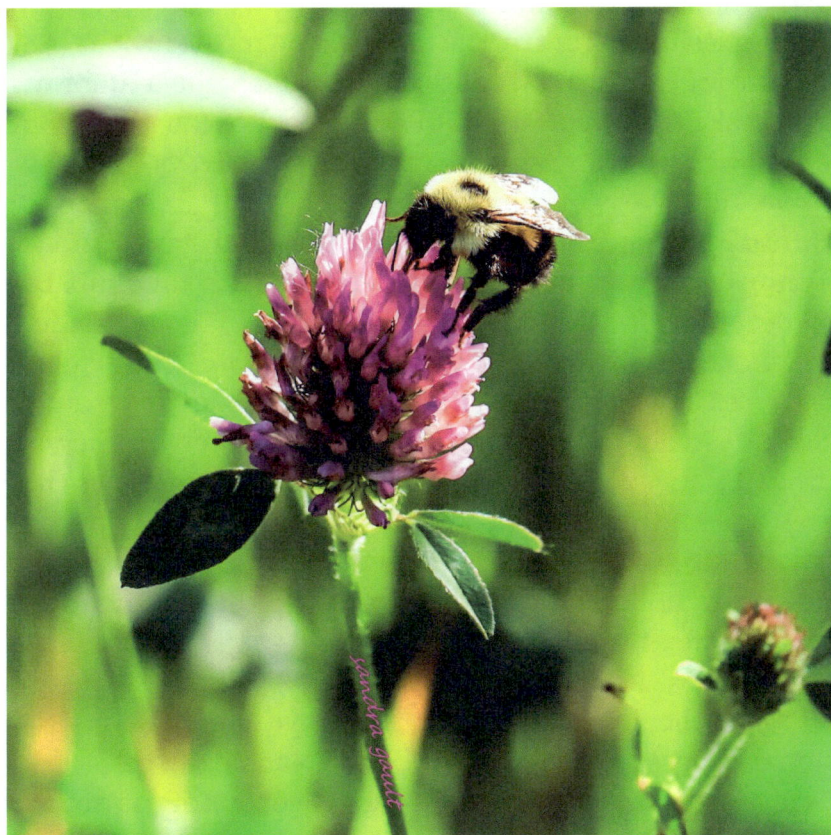

A TYPICAL DAY

Since the crash I live my life in 5-minute intervals. Let me explain. Have a shower; rest. Do the minimum possible to control the rat's nest on my head. Rest. Get dressed in comfortable clothing that does not irritate my skin. Take the bra off. Rest. Change socks because I cannot wear ones with any seams. My feet have always been sensitive, now with numbness, and pain, they are positively painful. To top it off I wiggle my toes and have restless, jumpy legs. Put soup on the stove. Rest. Burn the soup. Eat something out of a box. Nap. Put a load of laundry in; forget about it for the rest of the day. Order something online because I can't get out to shop. Nap or fall asleep in front of the TV? Avoid the phone ringing, and turn down the volume (it's always too loud). Open email and avoid ones that are too lengthy. I don't remember the last time I checked email. Put extra layers of clothing on; I was always warm, now I run hot and cold. I can never find the right warmth of throw for the couch. Too exhausted to get up and make a cup of tea. I must remember (ha, ha) to bring a mug of water to the couch so I don't get dehydrated. Put my National Geographic aside; maybe I can read next week.

On average it takes me 2 to 4 hours to get out of the door to an appointment or rare visits with friends.

The only thing I am capable of doing is to watch TV. Programs that have too much movement are now on the "can't watch" list. I open my eyes every 10 minutes or so and try to catch up on the show. After a few years of sleeping 18 to 20 hours a day, I am now only sleeping about 14 in total. It is not logical to me that I never feel rested. After leaving the TV on too much my TV stops functioning properly. Good thing it was under warranty. Years ago, I managed to connect the TV, stereo, DVD player, and VCR together, almost without reading instructions. Instructions? I toss them to the side now. Just like I feel my company and some friends did to me. I am better, I tell a friend, but she doesn't email back.

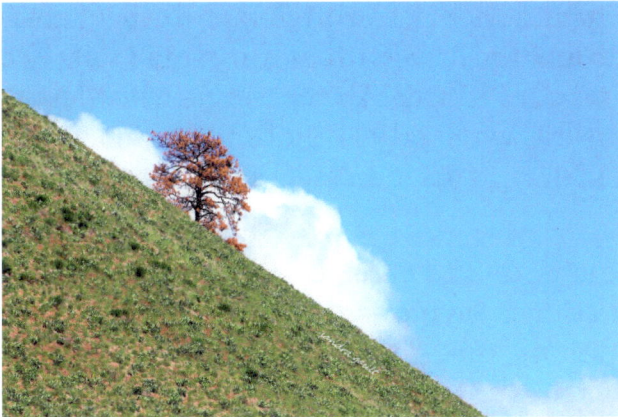

RELATIONSHIPS

Social butterfly, extravert, social and charity planner, vacation planner. Just a few words people used to say about me. I was almost completely bed-ridden for two years. Memory evades me of those first years; I am uncertain whether I had any social outings. I only remember what I wrote in my journal. I vaguely remember a good friend helping me walk into a coffee shop. I did not drive much the first year. I have been fiercely independent my whole life. I hated depending on family and friends for rides to appointments, so I often take a cab. I hated getting into a cab and the driver attempting small talk. I can't talk small. I wonder if it is like the movie One Flew Over the Cuckoo's Nest, when Jack Nicholson gets lobotomized? It's not that I felt cut off, I didn't feel anything other than fear.

My instructor says to pace ourselves and explain to others our limitations. Saying "no" never was, and continues not to be, a strong suit. Your friends and family will understand, he tells us. We do not live in a world where putting ourselves first is acceptable.

I feel guilt for not being at work, guilt for letting friends and family down, guilt for not responding to phone calls and emails, guilt for not helping others, guilt for not being a functioning member of society. I do not have the energy for anything. Being anywhere for more than a few hours puts me in bed for days. Not accepting invitations for an outing has become a new "thing". Even when promised I have to back out at the last minute. I feel like a shit. I hate talking now anyway. My stuttering, slurred speech, and confusion are killers to my confidence. Eventually I understand my body better when it gives me warning signs; a sudden severe headache, followed by vomiting and blackouts. I try to explain to friends and family that when I say I have to leave; it means running for the door and not the usual slow good-byes. For years I carry a vomit bag in my purse. I still carry antacids and Gravol.

Relationships and making friends always came easy. The only thing going on in my life is my worsening illness, so I don't have anything else to talk about. Where is the line on how much to talk about the illness and fear? There is no future; for me. What is going on in their lives is important, but I am unable to concentrate on what they are telling me. I was so much more; now I am nothing more than this mess of a body and brain. I was always the one to offer help; now I am the one needing help but I have an impossible time asking for it. Staying in the social loop? I was the organizer of the social outings. Communication is the key to nurturing relationships. I have always understood this.

I want to have a nap on the restaurant table, not be cheerful and conversational. Having always been an upbeat person, I think I confused people. "Don't complain" is what I hear in my head. One friend keeps asking why I am not back at work. I cheerfully (stupidly) try to tell her I am very ill. She stops talking to me. Six months later I send her a long email explaining that I am chronically ill and that I try to put my best face forward when seeing friends. I never hear from her again. Yes, I admit I have a "too nice" thing, and a need to please. It hurts to be rejected.

One year after the crash I meet a guy that also has fibromyalgia. We understand each other, we grew up in the same area, our parents are the same age, etc. We are alike. The joke was on me. I was in a relationship with a narcissist. He started slowly to show his true colors. When my father died, he did not console me. WTH! He was always right and started screaming when I did not agree with him. Eventually the emotional distress became overwhelming. His reactions became more and more volatile. One incident where the abuse became too much and I was sitting in front of the toilet vomiting, he stepped over me and did not say a word. There were to be many incidents like this. Narcicists only care about how you are contributing to their needs. I am done with romantic relationships.

(A personal poem)

Passages without distance.

Silence and vision.

Hearts unchanged by forever knowing, where

time is unrehearsed.

As the morning mist clears the dimension

becomes translucent.

What is revealed is the past and present – tears and laughter.

Winds blow strong.

But oneness remains.

Life? (A personal poem)

I'm not living the life I was meant to.
As imagined in my childhood.
Mine was to be full of light and clarity.
Dreams naturally fulfilled – the sun rarely setting on my imagination and desires.
Where and when did I stray from this path to happiness?
Or did it abandon me in purposeful thought?
Must I spend every moment of possible glory reaped in loneliness and desire?
If I abandon desire, abandon thought of rising above, will I then find peace?
Which path leads to enlightenment?
Which is more sorrowful to desire or not?

It feels like a death. Death of my former life. An ongoing death because it keeps getting worse. I don't know who I am anymore. All those years of work and studies! I have always been a planner. Now...what plans? Plan A, B...? Life happens when you are busy making plans, does not apply anymore. After 10 years still don't know what to do with myself. Give up, or suck it up? Neither! Now that I have time to think of the meaning of life, I am not any closer. What is it that evades me? I have tried so many things in an effort to find the things that define me. Was it a foolish quest? Does it matter I will likely go to my grave (well actually, I do not want to be buried) not knowing the answer(s)? Simplicity is unknown, as is tranquility.

Be forever young in your heart.
Be forever forgiving in your soul and the world will be young.

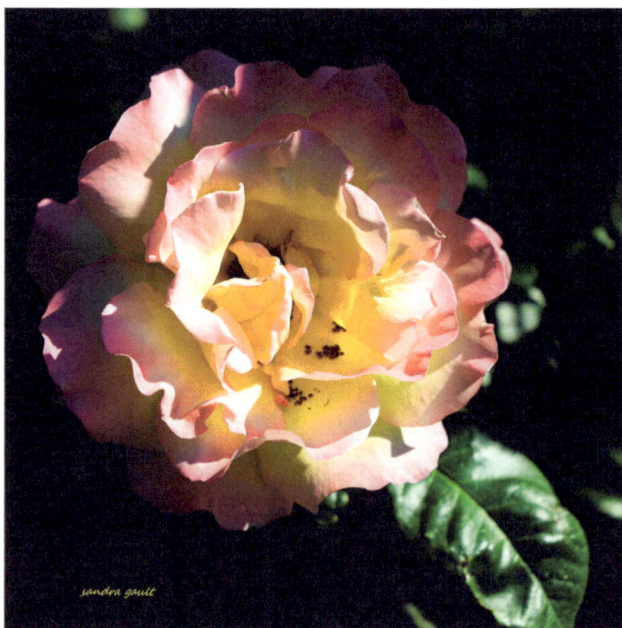

I wrote this a few years
before the crash:

ME –or at least the start (I apologize for the ultri-idealism):

I'm an idealist - I believe the world and our lives
are what we make them.

I believe the best in people (I smile at the world
and I expect them to smile back).

I love a sense of humor.

I love to talk and communicate. I like to know
what motivates people.

I think best when away from the world.

I believe in kindness, honesty and generosity.

Look at the world through the eyes of a child.

Making the best of anything that comes.

Not being too serious about myself.

Continuous desire to learn about the world
around me.

Standing up for what I believe in.

I believe everyone and everything is equal.

I am so many things, and yet feel as if I am nothing. We all
fade into nothing. I am deeply spiritual but again, what is
life without purpose? I don't believe in fate. All I have left is
who I am.

I have these annoying thoughts, without answers. I know I am running out of time! I have regret, heartache.

As long as you are not hurting someone, then live your life. Forget about expectations and traditions. Two years ago, I got a new tattoo of a lotus flower; through the mud I have crawled, but I am waiting for the full bloom. Recently at a meditation drum circle my spirit animal approached me. My warrior dragon is now tattooed on my leg next to the ancient Celtic symbol. A symbol of strength and mystical power. Only by sifting through the ordinary do we find what is true and beautiful.

Embrace your dreams
(A personal poem)

Pluck a dream from your surroundings,
And swallow it whole.
Let it essence take hold.
Release yourself to it.
Break free from chains that tie you to the
expected.
Let the light explode from your being in a brilliant
dance of joy.
To never let the darkness return.

I don't think I will ever stop looking. That is a definition of human intelligence in my belief. I want peace. I don't want my body to be touched (it hurts) and I have given up drinking. I rarely listen to music anymore. I need quiet. Being an almost life long vegetarian I am getting even pickier about what I put in my body, and the impact on the environment for that food. What I really need is an acreage where I can build a few small houses for my like-minded friends. There we can have our garden, enclosed areas for the doggies to run, peace and quiet.

I can see beyond (A personal poem)

I can see beyond.
Into a deeper world of love and gratitude.
A world of peaceful sharing and warm embraces.
A world of equals and balance.
I see it hiding under egos and pain.
Hide from your logic and let the rhythm of
peaceful breath guide your actions!

Who are you? - Space for reflection

I used to beat myself up on this subject. I think I know who I was. I certainly had strong feelings about it. I am embracing that life is changing more than it ever has. I don't have to explain to others who I am, or how I have changed.

Challenge: don't describe who you are!

AND THE FUN KEEPS COMING

I kept my old, favorite pair of hiking shoes; they still fit. I notice how the great support is making my walking more confident. I take this and a few other pairs of shoes to the podiatrist. After a walking assessment, he shows me how I am walking on the side of my left foot. After years of walking oddly because of my dislocated hip, I have developed a bunion. I am in serious need of orthotics to help my balance. Fitting shoes is an issue and orthotics are expensive. Walking is monumentally difficult if I have just taken Chloe for a walk, or I am overtired.

I ask my doctor for a handicap sticker; handicap! Why should I be embarrassed to be handicaped? It seems to be a combination of guilt and humiliation. People stare at me when I park in a reserved spot. I have been harassed by seniors for being in "their spot"! People don't understand how terrible and weak I feel. I have a problem getting into the store and need a cart for support. I want to wear dark glasses so nobody recognizes me. Fibromyalgia and chronic fatigue are invisible illnesses; to others.

After years of being immobile I developed more ailments; a lot more.

I developed high cholesterol because I relied on take out and frozen food. And while cooking is still too much work, I am eating simple, healthy food like humous and veggies.

Weight gain is a problem. It is creating high blood pressure. I have to take a tiny white pill every morning. I don't like it.

I used to think that Diabetes was either inherited or from eating too much bad food. I ate fairly well most of my life. Just after getting my puppy my doctor told me my health was in peril! Shit! What? A year after getting more active I was still pre-diabetic. The excess weight is the problem. Dieting with 2 chronic diseases (I hate the word disease) and a life-time of excessive stress is impossible. I stress eat; I always have. It's a long story. Extreme hunger happens with inadequate sleep and chronic stress. When the body is unreasonably tired it wants sugar. I also have an underactive thyroid, which makes EVERYTHING slower.

Fibromyalgia + chronic fatigue + chronic stress + underactive thyroid + walking problems + low iron + pre-diabetes = weight gain.

After two decades I finally get a real pain doctor. The local pain center has hired new doctors. My new doctor is so nice, and listens to everything I say. Listens! He goes over my history and meds and makes some medication adjustments. In my first few appointments I receive lidocaine injections in my neck and back. The ones in my neck make me dizzy, but there is less pain and tension. Signing my name is still hard from numb fingers. The brain only recognizes so much pain at a time. Something to do with electrical signals. It's a good thing, because now that my mid back is feeling a little better, the pain in other parts of my back feel worse. A few sleepless nights are worth it, because in general I am better.

Weather forecast: foggy, but clearing.

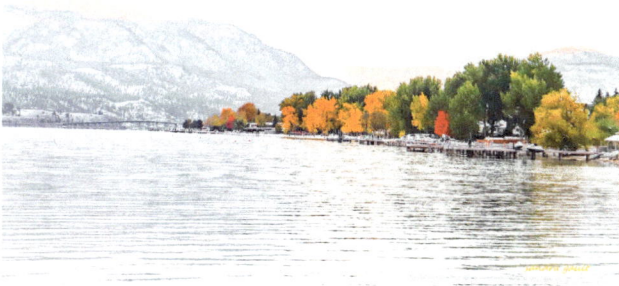

BEST REMEDIES

Five years after the crash I am able to read a little. The small stack of books I kept hold some interest. I have always dreamed of an old-fashioned library with a multitude of old books. Who published and read these books? Where did the books go on their travels? I start to believe I can continue expanding my knowledge. It is hard to get back into the reading habit/love, and I still get headaches if I read for too long.

Over the years I have come to understand that for me there is not one truth but many. I find that each conversation, television program, book and magazine touches on some part of our truth. The search for all of us is to put the pieces together that allow us the gift of understanding our self and our worth.

I need a dog in my life. The love and companionship are the best happy there is, for me. I start to search for a puppy; a small one that I can cuddle; a fuzzy one. I see several ads,; one for a Bichon. When I research the breed, they are perfect for me. I make inquiries and later that week I have a little fuzzy wuzzy.

OMG is she cute, and funny, and smart, and fuzzy, and...

My Chloe; the love of my life. Rolling around on the floor, getting up and down, feeding, cleaning, lots of cleaning, playing, cuddling. Its hard, really hard to move. For years I could not get off the floor if I fell. It takes a lot of effort and determination to move. I need to do this for her and for me. If I can't my future is bleak. If in my 50's I can barely move, then what kind of future do I have?

My Laughter is coming easily now because of Chloe, and everyone notices the change. When spring weather rolls around we go for longer and longer walks. It's a challenge. Walking was one of my "things". My balance is an issue, but we forge ahead. Buying sweaters are a challenge; they are either too feminine or masculine for Chloe. One friend suggests I sew on a frill at the end of the sweaters that are too short. LOL! She knows I hate pink and frills. I don't wear them and neither does my dog! I grew up outside playing sports, and games, picnics, building forts, playing with tree frogs, neighborhood hide and seek, searching for the elusive 4 leaf clover, making music with a thick blade of grass, riding my bike everywhere. Nothing better than a little fun and warm breeze on the face! Om.

There are dozens of parks close by, and I save the locations of easy ones on my phone. My little pup is a trooper. She is small, but strong and curious. She and I are loving the adventures. Every little trail offshoot we consider; I always did like the road less taken. Never have I been a follower. Walking in nature, with my little one, is meditative; my medicine.

My Chloe was socialized from day one. I take her everywhere I can, and she gets LOTS of attention. The online Bichon site has thousands of enthusiasts all over the world. Such sweetness, joy and silliness. It fills my heart. I need her like I need the air. The odd thing about being at home is that I finally get the rest I need. My somewhat wee 18-pound dog takes up most of the bed, of course. She sleeps in her soft, well padded crate, most of the night, but a few hours before the sun rises, she needs my company. A morning snuggle is the best way to start the day; it is calming. I need all the calm I can get. It is proven that rubbing a dog's tummy lowers blood pressure. Maybe I need more fuzzy wuzzies? Lol. Not going to happen. Chloe requires a lot of attention; and she gets it. Spoiled? No. Loved.

By that fall the strength in my body starts to come back, after 10 years of barely enough strength to hold a glass. Moving around in my various activities is a little easier. I still have to take a lot of rests between activities. Chloe and I have about the same amount of energy to walk, and we have a good nap when we get home. I will never feel like Hercules again. Feeling alive? Not quite.

Six months later a friend suggests a yoga class. It has been ten years. Knowing that yoga is not about how you are doing, but how you are feeling in your own body and space. It is gentle and enjoyable. It has been a year now since I started gentle Hatha classes. The work community I was so devoted to is gone, and now I have communities of doggie friends, and a lovely yoga group. I still need to look inward for answers, but I have more gentle earth creatures to support me on the path.

I have always loved photography; looking and analyzing, feeling and capturing. I have not given it much thought the past ten years. It sits gathering dust in the closet like many other things from the time before. How many people have asked me to take their family photos? If you had a family of birds, I may have considered it. I light up, and at the same time feel grounded when I am in nature. I don't need to concentrate on the breath, I am at one with nature's breath. I love an expanding landscape in front of me, and the tiny flower clinging to life on a gravel path. If nature is taking back its space with a barn or fence, that has interest. It all goes back to the earth. I grab my enthusiasm, because gathering energy is hard, along with puppy and camera and head outdoors. It feels like a chore to get up and out, but once out it is heaven, as does our long slumber back at home after. When my breath leaves me, I want my ashes to be placed in the ground with a tree to feed above. Energy continues on.

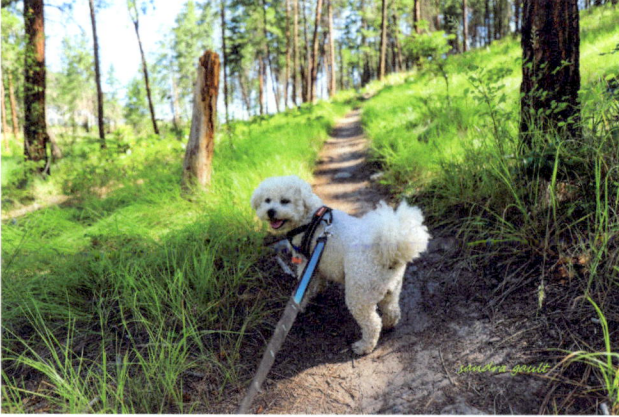

Don't panic - Space for reflection

I find myself panicking when symptoms change. Every-thing in our bodies change; constantly.

Time to breathe again. Fill the belly and let the ribs expand. Close your eyes.

Are there methods that work for you to calm yourself?

NOW

My world is puppy, walking, photography, TV, family and friends, and pondering life. As a younger person I embraced change. I lost most of my work friends. I have a new group of friends from the dog park. Recently I broke my ankle hiking. Wasn't wearing good enough hiking shoes. Ugh. After a day and a half in the hospital; after surgery, they send me home with crutches, walker, air boot and a bath seat. I am not allowed to even touch my foot on the ground for the first month. I got so depressed. I fought to get my mobility back. I buy a used knee scooter, and at least I can get around; sort of. I hire a dog walker for Chloe, but she doesn't want to walk without me. I cry when I see her leave. She has a massive zoomie when she gets home to me. I get some visits from friends, and a few take her to the dog park. She hates it. After a few weeks a friend takes us both to the park, with my knee scooter in tow. Joyous!

It is 8 weeks now, and I just had my first appointment with the physical therapist. I did lots of reading after I broke the ankle (not much else to do).

I got the okay from the surgeon at 6 weeks to start moving the ankle and weight bearing. YouTube is marvelous for learning exercises. My physio therapist said I was doing good. A little yoga will be good to get my flexibility and strength back. When I get home, I move all my mobility devices into the den, out of my sight. Thanks to walking Chloe in the past few years, and the determination to get better, I am stronger. Now, if only my sense of humor would return.

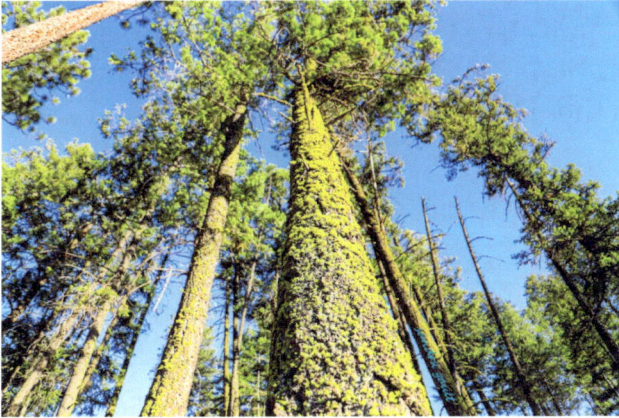

SUGGESTIONS

My communication style is collaborative. It is not my place to force my ideas on others. The suggestions below are based on my experiences. I hope you find them helpful.

Find a doctor to listen.

You must be your own advocate.

Find alternative, healthy full-body treatment.

Be knowledgeable and careful of drug side effects. That goes for herbs, and supplements. Be cautious of the combining prescription drugs and herbs/supplements. Learn the language from both sides of medicine.

Your intuition about your own body is your best guide.

Find support for physical and mental health.

Keep notes of changing symptoms. It is helpful for you and your doctors.

Keep notes to also see how far you have come.

Celebrate small successes.

Ditch the blame. I know what the final straw was, but it does me no good to dwell on it.

Try a little exercise even when you feel you can't. Yoga is

great for my body.

Find calm and listen to your body and heart.

You really are what you eat. Unless you cannot absorb the nutrients. Find out if this is also keeping you in a spiral of exhaustion.

Accept the new paradigm. Embrace the new life and be determined that it will have meaning and the opportunity to redefine or rediscover yourself.

Find some quiet time to be still and listen for the stirring of your soul.

Find Calm

Turn off the phones and find calm.

Only through calm reflection do we find balance.

One cannot listen to others or their own heart while speaking.

Take a walk; stare out the window; shut off the world and find what your heart and emotions are telling you. Stop worrying about everything.

Sit with the discomfort. This is where the answers are.

When you find calm the world around you becomes calmer.

Discover your strength and beauty – it's there.

Trust yourself. The answers are within. Believe that they will come.

Remove purpose from time and the mind will flow like

sweet water from an underground spring.

Mellow the depths of sorrow, and let the eyes reveal what the heart may shelter.

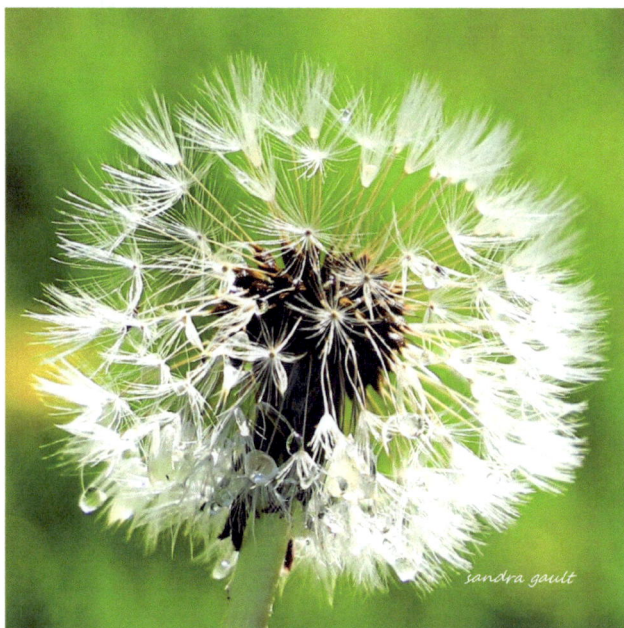

My life may be smaller, but for everyone life comes down to daily struggles to get through the mud and bloom in the wonderment of a lotus flower. Through the storm I have risen, again and again. To a more gentle life, and the love of a puppy.

Please feel free to make a list of your own ideas and wins on the road to feeling better.

*Live life consciously
(personal thoughts)*

Be true to your whole being.

Be kind to the wisdom of the earth.

Walk softly and breathe gently.

Speak with truth and quiet intelligence.

Be strong of heart and soft of gaze.

Feel deeply.

Be open to everything.

Don't judge.

Reach out to possibilities.

Smile often.

Experience moments of peace.

Never stop learning.

Keep company with your inner child.

Laugh honestly.

MY CHLOE

Check out my Instagram page to see more of my photos, taken on walks with My Chloe:

www.instagram.com/sandragaultphotography

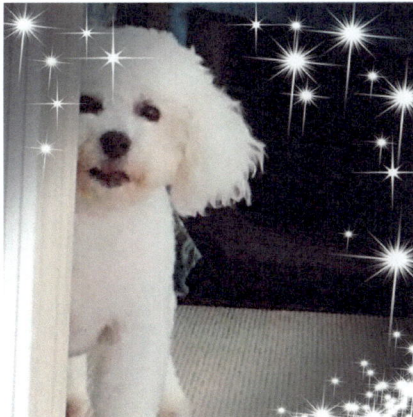

Manufactured by Amazon.ca
Bolton, ON